HOW TO MASTER A

FIT RICH LIFE

IN 15 DAYS!

TACTICAL ADVICE TO
CRUSH YOUR SELF-
LIMITING BELIEFS AND
CREATE YOUR OWN COME
BACK STORY

by
Jason and Pili Yarusi

How to Master a Fit Rich Life in 15 Days!

ISBN 978-0-578-23899-9

Printed in USA by 48HrBooks (www.48HrBooks.com)

TABLE OF CONTENTS

INTRODUCTION AND PREPARATION

"You begin to fly when you let go of self-limiting beliefs and allow your mind and aspirations to rise to greater heights." – Brian Tracy

Not where you thought you would be at this stage of your life?

Want more and know you can accomplish more but just can't seem to break out of your current state?

If your answer is "yes," then good news!

We are very excited to bring this book to YOU to give you tactical steps to eliminate excuses and become a difference maker. Isn't it time to overcome your doubt and create winning beliefs that will prepare you to take on the world one giant leap at a time?

This book will help you achieve your goals, heal your most difficult relationships and do what is right for you and your loved ones. This book will help you break out of your routine and become more successful in your daily life. The steps here will give you the tools to overcome any barrier to success and never look back.

This is it! The ultimate Life Action Plan in 15 days.

What is this book really about?

Create your own story. Run your own business. Conquer your fears and have a little fun along the way!

By removing your self-limiting beliefs, ANYTHING becomes possible and this book will show you just how we do it.

We always have the ability to control our thoughts and actions and what we do and say. And it starts with making the decision *right now* to do so.

It takes effort to establish the right practices and habits to release your true potential. What follows are the steps we use and continue to use to break our own boundaries and continue to push forward towards a Fit, Rich Life.

Who Are We?

We are Jason and Pili Yarusi, active Real Estate Syndicators and Investors. In 2016 we founded Yarusi Holdings, a multifamily investment firm currently with over 800 apartment units under management. Our firm repositions properties through operational efficiencies, moderate to extensive renovations and complete re-branding. We also host "The Jason and Pili Project," a podcast that sets the foundation for building mental fortitude, growing wealth and improving health. Our monthly meet up, The New Jersey Multifamily Formula Club has over 2,000 members and focuses on Real Estate Syndication.

Beyond real estate, we spend incredible amounts of time with our three young kiddos Luke, Lily, and Leo. Watching them grow and discover all that life has to offer.

We are avid workout enthusiasts. Jason has found a love for kettlebell workouts and long distance running, completing to date a number of Ultramarathons with the longest being 101 miles. Pili has found her passion for running, pushup challenges and cross functional activities that involve playing with the kiddos.

We love helping others improve and solidify their futures with our Fit, Rich, Life growth and leadership coaching that provides tactical actions steps to building a fulfilling life.

We wrote this book together but sometimes Jason wrote certain parts, and Pili wrote others. We will try our best to let you know when we switch it up.

It is our sincere hope that you greatly benefit from our work together in order to assist you to get a Fit, Rich Life!

In order to be a success in life, you have to take action. Before we get into the actual steps for each day, follow the following action step and don't wait!

The universe LOVES speed...

ACTION STEP:

Text us, "FitRichLife," at +1 (908) 224-6876

Introduce yourself and let us know why you picked up this book!

DAY 1:
DEFINE FULFILLMENT

You were put on this earth to be special. You were not put here to be average. Now it's time to start acting like it again. Sit up taller, be proud of yourself and know you are the person you wish you were.

The goal of this day is to establish what you really want.

Do you want more time? A happy family? Money? Better relationships? Each one of these and more?

Why?

What is it that achieving this will mean to you?

What will achieving this give to you?

And... if you don't achieve it, what will happen?

A goal is in reach when it is significant enough to you. Too many times we set a goal based on something that sounds good or looks great on social media but we have no emotional tie to it.

In reality, if we don't know why we want something, truly want it, then it really won't matter if we get it or not. Nor will our journey have any purpose.

"Would you tell me, please, which **way** I ought to go from here?"

"That depends a good deal on where you want to get to," said the Cat.

"I don't much care where—" said **Alice**.

"Then it doesn't matter which **way** you go," said the Cat.

About ten years ago I (Jason) felt lost. I was angry – not necessarily at anyone or anything but it was a combination of not truly being in control of my feelings and not being comfortable in my own skin to truly discuss my thoughts with anyone. I was angry at my situation and I found ways to blame others for my insecurities.

But after distancing my relationships and failing at my current venture, I learned that only I was in control and responsible for where I was. And when I was able to reel my mind in from the fog and look only at my current day and not worry about tomorrow, I was able to start making progress towards being a better me.

In other words, I took full responsibility for my life and started to live in the present moment. I stopped all regret for the past and all worry about the future.

And that's what we want for you to do for yourself too.

The following action steps are going to help you to figure out what you truly want in life by asking yourself some probing questions.

Here they are.

ACTION STEP:

Get out a pen and some paper and write down your answers to the following questions.

What words come to mind when you think of your perfect day?

Relaxing, challenging, creative, loving, enthusiastic, fulfilling? Don't hold back. What are the first things you think of?

Now, answer this Question: What Does a perfect day look like to you? Do not censor your thoughts. Write for at least 10 minutes. The key is to be as descriptive as possible.

Where are you? What is the weather like? What does the air smell like? Who is with you? What are you wearing? What are you doing at each stage of the day?

Be honest. You are writing this for you. If you short-change the answers, you will only be limiting yourself.

DAY 2:
WHAT DRIVES YOU?

"You must expect great things of yourself before you can do them." – Michael Jordan

What drives you to be better, do better? What drives you to be the best version of yourself?

When you expect great things out of yourself, your subconscious mind will work silently in the background in order to create that reality for you.

But another question we want you to answer is, *WHY ARE YOU DOING WHAT YOU DO?* What drives you?

Right now is a great time to find out and establish your WHY.

Your "why" is whatever it is that you value the most that will get you motivated and inspired to take action. Your "why" will help you to get up in the morning.

For me (Pili), my systems get me up. I know that in order to be my best self for my family *I need to take care of me first.* As of right now, I roll out of bed at 5 am and on to my yoga mat. I do my meditation practice and do 45 minutes of yoga… The kiddos usually find me around 6 still on my yoga mat… and then I jump into the rest of my day!!!

Who makes you do what you do?

I make the choice to wake up and take on my day. It is my responsibility. Right now, however, today was difficult.

I slept in a bit because of a pinched nerve in my back and did a shortened Yoga practice. I wasn't able to play with my kids or give my husband my full attention because I was focused on the discomfort. It took me awhile to decide to take on my day. I was going to skip my run and pushups but I didn't and I am glad. I forced myself outside and I came back home with more energy because I had made the decision to show up instead of letting the morning take me down.

What does financial freedom mean to you?

For me, it's not having to worry about my children's financial future. We will teach them to be self-sufficient and they will also know the power of generational wealth because we will continue to build it. We will create servant leaders and we will teach our children how to use money correctly and how to manage their finances correctly.

How does a fulfilling life look for you?

At this moment, my youngest is napping peacefully in his bed. The older two are playing happily with their Daddy – and it is the middle of the day on a Wednesday. Jason and I are rich with TIME – we have set up our lives in such a way that we can use more of our time for ourselves, each other and our children.

What is your BIG WHY?

Jason, our children, our family and those who are within our circle are my biggest why. But also, keeping myself fit and fulfilled is very important too so that I may serve them fully.

"It's not enough to have lived. We should be determined to live for something." —Winston S. Churchill

ACTION STEP:

Answer these questions. Be real and honest with yourself:

- What gets you up in the morning?

- Who makes you do what you do?

- What is the drive behind reading this book?

- What does financial freedom mean to you?

- How does a fulfilling life look for you?

- What is your BIG WHY?

DAY 3:
SEE YOUR VISION

WHAT IS A VISION BOARD?

Vision boards are motivational tools to help you gain a clear understanding of what your goals are and what you want your life to look like. They can be for your personal life, professional life, or both.

WHY DO I NEED A VISION BOARD?

You want to create a vision board and put it somewhere you will see every day so you can remind yourself and physically see what your goals are. When you see what you want every day, you reach your subconscious mind and engage the law of attraction. The law of attraction states that positive thoughts bring positive experiences into your life. However, the same holds for negative thoughts.

HOW DO I CREATE MY VISION BOARD?

First, you want to take five minutes (set a timer) and really think about what you want. Think about what you want your life to look like. Close your eyes and visualize it. Really focus and concentrate on the details – the more detailed, the better.

Now that you have an understanding of what your goals are and what you want your life to look like, go ahead and find images, quotes and pictures that match and go along with these goals. Basically, it can be whatever you want. This is unique to you and your goals so get as creative as you want with it.

Make sure that wherever you put together your vision board, that you are able to edit and change it. You don't want it to be permanent, because sometimes our goals and motivation changes over time. So, you want to be able to take things off and put things on as you go along.

Next, you want to put it somewhere you will see it every day. The best place is somewhere you will see it when you wake up and before you go to bed. If you have it on a computer or digital frame, have it running as a screensaver so you can see it easily.

HOW TO USE YOUR AMAZING NEW VISION BOARD

Look at your vision board daily and every morning as you get ready for the best day of your life. Or, you could look at it in the afternoon during a particularly hard moment. And then, look at it in the late evening time in order to set yourself up to dream awesome dreams.

VISUALIZE the items on your board. Make them REAL – as if you are there. If you added words to your vision board, what do they mean to you? How do they make you feel?

Use this Daily and as often as you need it. BUT REMEMBER...

YOUR VISION IS NOTHING WITHOUT ACTION!

For me (Jason), it took a car and a bike to make me really identify what I needed. I left work one Saturday night after midnight and sped off on my fixed gear bike down the westside highway in New York City and across west 28th street. I was feeling alone, like I was working harder than others around me but we were all at the same place.

With the warm breeze of a July night, I turned off of 28th street and down 2nd avenue, watching a light ahead of me turn green. Out of the corner of my eye I caught a flash and next thing I remember is being bounced off the windshield of a car and flying through the air. I smacked the pavement with my limp body and rose slowly and unsteadily to my feet. The person in the car pulled up to me and asked, "Are you okay?" Body bloody, arm hanging to the ground and bike mangled I think I replied, "I think so..." and the car slowly rolled forward and then quickly took off.

I looked behind me at the racing cars on 2nd avenue beginning to steam ahead from the green light and luckily, two Norwegian guys and a girl raced into the street and helped me hobble gingerly to the side of the road.

Over the course of the night, I had a long time to look truly inside of myself. I was lucky to be alive and I made a decision to no longer waste time bringing my own life down. It didn't happen immediately, but I started to look at my days and my time differently. I began to slow down when it was needed and always kept looking forward towards a vision of what my future would be.

The moral of the story is, don't let the moments pass you by! Appreciate every single moment that you have on planet earth – none of us really know how long we have. This is why it's so important to find your vision and create your journey.

When you have a near-death experience, it puts EVERYTHING into perspective...

ACTION STEP:

Create your vision board!

DAY 4:
THE ALOHA MINDSET

"The world will turn to Hawai'i as they search for world peace because Hawai'i has the key... And that key is aloha!" - Aunty Pilani Paki

Want your perfect day? Let's bridge the gap between where you are and where you will be.

Are you sad, depressed, confused, unsatisfied, or disconnected? We all face these at some points in our life, during our weeks and our days. Labeling this and understanding what drives these feelings is massively important. Why? Because being present with your state of mind allows you to take control of your feelings. You do control your feelings and what you do about them. Knowing where you are is the best way to road map the steps you need to take to move from depressed to excited, confused to determined or disconnected to fulfilled.

Aloha!!! Pili here – A revered Native Hawaiian poet, author and spiritual guide, Aunty Pilani Paki said "The world will turn to Hawai'i as the search for world peace because Hawai'i has the key... And that key is Aloha!" In the paragraphs that follow you will find an acronym that Jason and I created together from our morning routine and how we try to conduct ourselves everyday – with ALOHA! But I was not the first to create an acronym for ALOHA - Aunty Pilani created one of the most profound meanings of ALOHA:

A - Akahai - Kindness expressed with a feeling of tenderness

L – Lokahi – Unity expressed with a feeling of harmony

O – Oluolu – Agreeable expressed with a feeling of pleasantness

H – Haahaa – Humility expressed with a feeling of modesty

A – Ahonui – Patience applied with perseverance.

This Acronym, also known as the Aloha Chant, has inspired millions and was the ignition for the Aloha Spirit Bill by the Hawaiian Legislature in 1986 and states, "The ALOHA Spirit was the working philosophy of native Hawaiians and was presented as a gift to the people of Hawai'i."

Here is the Acronym that Jason and I created:

CREATE ALOHA BY CHANGING YOUR BODY, LANGUAGE and MIND. I find when I start my day with Aloha, Aloha carries me through everything!

FIVE STEPS TO BRING A.L.O.H.A. INTO YOUR DAY

A - Awakening. Get out of bed! Brush your teeth, drink a glass of water, splash water on your face, and make your bed… Do anything to tell your body and mind that "It is time to start this day!" This should take you less that 3 minutes. These are the first moments of your day. Spend them awakening the mind and body. Need prep for this? Place you phone (and alarm) across the room, preferably in the bathroom. That way you can turn off your alarm and splash your face with water.

L - Love. These next 5-10 minutes are spent on meditation, gratitude and affirmations. Whether it be silent or guided meditation, prayer or silence, use this time to reset and start the day fresh. Be kind to yourself and be thankful for what you have and grateful for everything around you. Speak affirmations that lend to who you are becoming. Speak in the present. "I live a life filled with Aloha…"

O - Opportunity. If you can see it, you can believe it! Set your actionable goals for today and big overarching goals for the future. Then spend the next 10 minutes visually mirroring what the outcome will look like. Be as detailed as possible, so real that you can taste and smell it.

H - Health. Use this time to get moving. Exercise, stretching, physical expression or a combination of each. I (Pili) pound my chest and tickle my belly to enliven my body and to bring a little bit of silliness into my morning before exercising. Follow healthy eating habits and routine to fully engage and nourish your body throughout your productive day. Neither Jason nor I are nutritionists but one suggestion – cut out/back on processed food and drink more water. I have found that by simply cutting alcohol out of my daily life, my life has brightened immeasurably! Jason and I also practice intermittent fasting: We only eat between the hours of 8am – 6pm. This gives our system time to work and we have found that we sleep better when we don't eat late.

A - Aspire. Find greatness in your surroundings or the available lessons from others. Spend this time to read a self-development book or autobiography. Use this knowledge to catapult yourself forward. Learn the lessons others have endured to reach their highest potential. Once you reach your next level, use what you have found to help others also achieve the same.

I (Pili) slowly started sprinkling these in little by little each morning. At first, I felt silly and awkward doing these and was doing them more because I thought I should be, not understanding that I needed to be. Once I let go and gave myself permission to fully engage with my morning routine, I started to reap the massive benefits. Now my morning is like clockwork. This lets me control the beginning of my day, which gives me guidance to take on the rest of the day. Is everyday perfect? Not with three kids under six... But for most days, I make my morning routine a priority and it has been a huge reason for my success.

My Current Routine:

Wake up and have two glasses of water and make a cup of coffee with almond milk.

If I wake up early enough I will immediately go into a 45 minute Ashtanga Yoga practice or I will Meditate for ten minutes. I usually use Priming from Tony Robbins, the CALM APP or if I happen to be in a park or by the beach – anywhere in nature – I just sit in silence. Regardless, I focus on my breath the entire time.

This is followed by five minutes of visualization.

After this I say three affirmations ten times each.

Next, I spend at least five minutes stretching and once Jason is home from his run, I finish with a 45-minute run. I always take an empty bag with me to pick up trash along the way.

Then, I get back and welcome the time with my family and have breakfast.

And finally, I shower and get after my day.

ACTION STEP:

Take charge of your life! Create Your Aloha Mindset today. Take five minutes to write down what your perfect day looks like! When that is complete, write down three affirmative sentences that describe who you are in this perfect day. Only three sentences. Use the most creative and descriptive words you can. What is the fire that is going to light the candle, the fuel that drives the machine, the passion that encompasses your soul? WHY do you want this?

Pili's affirmations:

"I am living a life FILLED WITH ALOHA!"

"I share this ALOHA with all I encounter. This is my personal mission."

"I find ALOHA everywhere I go. I fill my SPIRIT FULL OF ALOHA from all that I encounter."

Next, see how you can sprinkle in a little ALOHA into your morning.

DAY 5:
TAKE SIMPLE AND SMART ACTION

"Life is complicated, fragile and difficult." What would happen if we stopped using this excuse? What if we told ourselves that this life we have right now is our only life? Perhaps it is best then to slow it down so we can build the speed back up.

Slow down to go fast is a motto that a lot of long-lasting companies adhere to. Sometimes you have to stop the chaos, even if it's costly, to let the dust settle so you can see what balls you are actually juggling and then astutely choose which balls to let drop.

The first step is to identify the spaces you adhere to in your life. Your list may comprise of marriage, parenting, adventure, fitness, hobbies, health and work. Identify which part of each area brings you the most joy and which part brings the most pain. Identify both no matter how difficult. The key is to decipher the joy from the pain and then find a bridge that leads you constantly to the joy in each space when you find yourself being pulled towards the pain.

Next, chunk each category into at most five mini-categories and prioritize these spaces. Family may split into spouse, children, siblings and parents. Health may dissect into workouts, eating habits and sleep routine. Then look at how all of these spaces correlate. Remember there is never a perfect balance. If you put all your attention into family, your job may suffer or if you fully focus on business your health may deteriorate. The key here is to find your joy and then commit to being fully committed when you are working in each space. In other words, don't be on work calls when playing with your kids. Or, don't feel bad if you are out to dinner with your partner and not working on the book you want to write. When you are in each space working towards your joy, be present and be fully engaged. Our focus today is finding a smart goal for each space.

"If we compete with ourselves and not with others, then it does not matter who is behind us or ahead of us; our goal is to become and achieve all we are capable of being and doing, and this becomes the measure of our satisfaction." — Myles Munroe

HOW TO CREATE SMART GOALS

SMART is an acronym for
S - Specific
M- Measurable
A- Attainable
R- Relevant
T- Timely

S - Specific

"I want more money!" Ok. Here is a dollar! That's more money…

THE UNIVERSE WANTS YOU TO BE SPECIFIC. You need to define your goal with as many minute details as possible. "I will net $10,000.00 US dollars a month by buying 15 cash flowing properties in San Antonio by January 30 2021." Now that's specific! The universe gets the clear picture, and along with your subconscious mind, will work to create that reality.

M- Measurable

We use the principles in the "12 Week Year" by Brian Moran. Each goal you choose should have a series of 3-5 measurable actions. Stop thinking of accomplishments based on years. Why can't you achieve four years worth of goals in one year's time?

A- Attainable

"I want $10,000.00 right this second." For most of us, this is not attainable. But take it a step further... Your goal(s) should be realistic. Look at this example: "I will net $10,000.00 US dollars a month by buying 15 cash flowing properties in San Antonio by January 30 2021." This is attainable by learning, implementing and doing the work required.

R- Relevant

If you want to get into Real Estate Investing, then your goal should be tuned into Real Estate Investing.

Not Relevant: "I will net $10,000.00 US dollars a month by buying 15 cash flowing properties in San Antonio by January 30 2021 but I may try dropshipping, trade Bitcoin or become a paid writer instead." You learn by doing but lack of focus keeps you where you are.

RELEVANT: "I will net $10,000.00 US dollars a month by buying 15 cash flowing properties in San Antonio by January 30 2021 that are built after 1980 and are at least four to eight units each."

T- Timely

Give your goal a deadline. Give each action a deadline. Define what will happen if you reach this goal. What will happen if you don't?

The first-known use of the term SMART Goals occurred in the November 1981 issue of Management Review by George T. Doran.

Jason and I used to work for this amazing couple, John and Angela Krevey. Captain John used to like to bring up a story about me from the first year I worked for him.

This was 2003 - Chelsea, NYC - This is before gentrification and beautification hit this area of the city. The Hudson River was a dangerous place to be at night and I worked in a bar on a barge docked at Pier 23. This was The Frying Pan or Pier 63 Maritime.

It was a busy night. I worked in the boat bar with Dave and Nick and I had placed 5 other bartenders outside in the Barge bar. At this time The Frying Pan was not the well-oiled day time drinking paradise it is today – nope. This was a dive bar/dance hall/artist haven all run by a Lightship Captain.

I have many stories of this amazing place, but let's save that for another day…

The story I want to tell you is this…

The night was wrapping up and we'd had a monster night - probably 10 deep at each register and the music was going off! I don't remember who was there that night but they'd brought in over 3000 folks who wanted to let loose and have some fun.

While we were closing up, Dave and I stayed to clean and I sent Nick to the back to count tips because he'd been working a double and needed a break.

Less than 3 minutes later, Nick came rushing back to me shouting, "They stole the tips!"

I didn't know what "they" looked like, but I knew there were only two ways off the boat – jump in the water, or go off the ramp. I saw them running and decided to take off after them.

(Note here: This is 2003 - I am a 125 lbs, 23 year old, I hate running, don't like going to the gym but I did yoga to keep fit. In other words, not the person you want running after two large men who look like they play football!)

But I made the decision and took action. I yelled past the outside bartenders. I yelled at the security guards who let them out. I yelled across West Side Hwy. I yelled past the strip bar that was at the corner. I yelled past a guy talking to some folks by his car. And I kept running.

Thank goodness that last guy in his car was an Undercover NYPD. He followed me, drove past me and caught the guy. One of them at least.

So, why did I tell you this story? For one, it's pretty funny. Two, it started me on a journey of personal health, wellness and kick-assery. The point is that inspiration can come from anywhere!

Here were my new SMART goals:

S- Specific goal. Become a runner and learn to defend myself.

M- Measurable. Run 10 miles three days a week. Take a Jeet Kune Do class at least two days a week. Make sure that class has measurable guidelines to track progress. I also had an accountability partner who would meet me to workout, get me used to gym life and take me kayaking every so often in the Hudson River.

A- Attainable. See above. All attainable.

R- Relevant. I want to defend myself. Super relevant.

T- Timely. I started this in the Summer of 2003 and continued until I left NYC for LA in 2005. This had no time stamp but every month I would notice the difference in my strength and ability.

ACTION STEP:

Pick a goal.

Write it out exactly how I have done it above. This will make your Goal more real and attainable.

Commit to that goal for the next five days. When it becomes routine, choose another space and repeat.

DAY 6:
CHANGE YOUR FOCUS

Are your current daily actions good or bad? Are you afraid if you try something it won't work and are too fearful of failure to try, or are you overly concerned about what others will think? Think long term. You are now in control your thoughts, feelings, actions and what you say.

We've grown too comfortable – conditioned to a life where we still feel the human instinct of survival ingrained in each of us, yet, there aren't any saber tooth tigers chasing after us and meals arrive at our doorstep with the touch of an app.

Regardless, so many of us are unhappy. Very unhappy.

Even as our world has been getting more and more comfortable, we can still experience pain in our hearts from dreaded loneliness, or some other negative thought, feeling or event. We accept that our phones will let us know when something is amiss, or social media gives us our value by seeing how many people like our post. Why have we let this happen?

Instead of relishing the opportunity to find what we want, we still rely on our primal instincts to suspend our emotions within a state of survival.

Data shows that scientifically we are living in the best years ever... We are blessed to be in a world where opportunity exists and the ability to change our circumstances is forever possible.

So, what is it? What is holding *us* back from finding fulfillment? What keeps us up at night unable to find our purpose?

We have found these three things play a huge role in defining our happiness both positively and negatively.

1. Lack of Commitment

We lack commitment not because we didn't "want" to but because we hadn't found focus and meaning to what we were doing. Being that this is the greatest time, rarely are we put in a position where if we don't do "X," it will lead to some massive upheaval in our life like our family starving. So, we wait and wait and wait some more to do just the minimum because, what's the worst that can happen?

What are we waiting for? Well, the right time of course – a magical moment when the heavens will shine down and announce that "NOW" is the time and now is our moment to get going. I truly believe this moment does happen but when it does, guess what? We aren't ready, because we haven't prepared for the moment to arrive and it's wasted, because what is being given to us is well above what we are ready to receive and achieve.

2. Try Once and Give Up

Equally on par with lacking commitment is our inability to face rejection, difficulty and uncertainty. We try what we just saw on YouTube and when we don't have results in five minutes, our response is either "I knew this wouldn't work" or "That person is so lucky to start at the right time" or "They must have gotten lucky" or one of a number of other generic responses.

Well how about "We didn't put in the work." Nothing good comes easy. While we know this, it doesn't make doing without receiving a quick reward or instant gratification any easier.

We have come to expect that if we want it, we get and that's happiness. Except that's not how it works and when we get smacked in the face with reality, it comes down to how committed we are in #1 – to know if we are actually going to make it over the hump to the next step.

3. Caring what others think

"Always be yourself and have faith in yourself. Do not go out and look for a successful personality and try to duplicate it." – Bruce Lee

This has stopped each of us at some point in our life, whether it was trying a new thing, asking someone out or changing courses in our life. We all have not done something because of what "Joe" may think of us.

Well, here's the truth about "Joe" – he's not thinking about you, because "Joe" has too many things on his plate to worry about you too and even if he was thinking about you, judging you, so what?

Truth is you may look stupid at first trying something new. I don't know many people who want to horseback ride that just get on a horse and ride off like John Wayne. Imagine if babies thought like this, they would never walk. So, who are we to judge others and let others judge us?

Want more. Want to be more. Want to get more done.

It's as simple as:

Commit.

Don't quit.

Stop caring what others think.

When I was 17 (this is Jason) my girlfriend was killed in a car accident. This capped 4 years of tragic events that also included my best friend being killed in a boating accident, a teammate killed in a car accident and a friend I had grown up with committing suicide. To say I was lost was an understatement. At my girlfriend's funeral, I had in my mind that I should be crying but I couldn't find those emotions and I was just empty.

For years, I couldn't find a tear until my first child was born and I felt this wave of feelings that I honestly couldn't identify. At 17, I was making a lot of important decisions with the next step in my life but I felt like my worth was lost and I didn't deserve so I simply took what came to me. From schooling to relationships to the future, I stopped putting drive behind it with the fear that if I cared too much, it would somehow again be abruptly taken away.

No plan, no perfect day and no future expectations. It took a moment of realization some years later to understand this basic thought, "No matter what happened yesterday, the key to my future is in my decision today." I chose to craft the life I wanted and focus on only the positive and no longer let the negative be the conversation driver. This has and is what has brought me to be the man I am today.

ACTION STEP:

Commit yourself to 15 days straight of continued action. This is for you to become who you already are and now it's time to show yourself who's in charge. Repeat to yourself five times "I am strong. I am healthy. I choose happiness. I am successful."

DAY 7:
BREAK THE PATTERN

"One day, in retrospect, the years of struggle will strike you as the most beautiful." - Sigmund Freud

Go right when it says go left. Take time to take massive deliberate action. You no longer have problems; you are the Chief Problem Solver.

A change of a routine can be difficult, enlightening, game-changing or frustrating – it just really depends at how you look at it.

Here is a list of things you can do daily to keep yourself on track and not get lost down a social media or Netflix rabbit-hole.

1. Keep a routine to your clock. Don't change your sleep pattern. Change what you do with the time when you are awake.
2. Get up and move. The simple act of going to work provides movement. Make sure to fill this gap with simple exercises like walking up and down stairs.
3. Work in blocks. If you are home with family, don't try to work through them. Block time to maximize your production.
4. Smile. This is so powerful and can alter the current state you're in. If you are on the phone and smile

while you are talking, the person you are speaking with can actually sense this.

5. Max out your calendar. The time spent commuting is ripe for the taking to tackle that passion project you have always thought about – even if it's listening to podcasts to learn about what you want to do.

6. Get unstuck. Ask how you can help daily. Get out of your own head by focusing on others.

7. Don't worry. Prepare. Worrying is time wasted not getting prepared and what you worry about will not be anywhere close to what actually happens.

Life is as we make it and our perception does become our reality.

It is key to create a new pattern to transition from and not look for extreme change. Radical transformation is not sustainable. That is why New Year's Resolutions fail over 85% of the time each year. The process has not been built. The desired change is too foreign to our routine.

Going from sitting on the couch to running a marathon in a week won't work, but what if you started with a 10 minute walk each day? Studies show that setting small goals that you can easily meet and continuing them is better than setting goals that are too hard to attain.

Completing a to-do list with 100 items on it is overwhelming, but what if you make the decision to pick the three most critical tasks to your day and to accomplish just those?

That is a recipe for success.

As you build up, you may go from a 10-minute walk to a 15-minute jog to an hour spin class and your mind and body will enjoy the process and not dread the next step. This is your life now and this is what you do. Not what you have to do but what you get to do. Create life habits, not fads.

I like drinking beer (this is Jason :) and back almost 20 years ago, I started having a few beers a day and sometimes would overindulge. The trend carried on until about 18 months ago that I would drink daily. It had been years since I drank to be drunk, but I drank a few beers each and every day and then would crush myself with a workout the following morning, punishing myself for the night before. I started realizing that my reactions were slowing and my thoughts were foggy, but I thought I needed this because it was what I do. But then I realized that if I drank two beers a day at an average of 154 calories a beer, I was adding an astounding 32 pounds of weight to work off each year. Over 20 years that's over 600 pounds! Not to mention the wasted money. For me, luckily, I had Pili. She never criticized me but instead, just helped me sculpt better decisions and together we made a plan where I eventually broke that habit for a week, then a month, then months. I still like a good beer but now, I enjoy it and don't consider it my routine. We are in control of our decisions whether we are making good or bad ones!

ACTION STEP:

Smile. Then look at your day and create 5 ten-minute blocks where you will completely dedicate yourself to the task at hand. For that ten minutes, you are laser focused on the task at hand and nothing will break you away. This will create a habit of dedication and commitment that you will use to grow your ability to engage and conquer what's ahead.

Bonus Round:

It's time to test your progress so far. Scale the following as needed, but this is a stress test to establish where you are and in a month do it again to see how far you come. We repeat this on the 15th of every month and it takes only 10 minutes.

The 'Max' mind and body stress test

Complete these 10 actions in 10 minutes not exceeding 1 minute on any step

- Wall sit 60 secs

- Breath hold as long as able

- Push-ups all out 60 seconds

- Words in a minute that start with (pick one each time) *th, wo, re, ph, mi, de, re, sa, pe, bo*

- Plank 60 secs

- Say This Tongue Twister as many times as possible;
  "Peter Piper picked a peck of pickled peppers
  A peck of pickled peppers Peter Piper picked
  If Peter Piper picked a peck of pickled peppers
  Where's the peck of pickled peppers Peter
  Piper picked?"

- 2 minutes visualize graphically your perfect house

- Bear walk 60 seconds

- Read a page out loud speaking loudly every fifth word

- Free squats 60 seconds

DAY 8:
UNDO THE "THINKING ABOUT IT" HABIT

"It is never too late to be what you might have been"
– George Eliot

At 41 years old, for me, Jason, there are days when I look back and think, "how did I get here?"

I don't mean that in either a negative or a positive way – I just mean that life hardly ever turns out the way we imagine. If I look back to when I was 13 or 22, life turned out a lot different than I would have ever thought.

When I truly look at my life and look at what I have and what I have accomplished, I have found it's been breaking bad mental habits that have gotten me to where I am, but also mental roadblocks have kept me where I am.

Now that may sound like I am talking out of both sides of my mouth, but when you dig down deep, we are only able to ever be what our mind can grasp.

From my own experiences I have found there are generally *four blocks* that keep you where you are.

#1) Needing to know more before I proceed

••••

From starting a side project to trying a new hobby, the need to know everything before beginning separates the pack. Do and have, or ponder and have not. The truth is, you will never know everything and the greatest learning experiences are in the doing, not the thinking about doing.

2) What will others think about me if I do this....

This was stated prior but such a showstopper that it needs to be repeated. So many times, we don't start because of what others may think. It's amazing that we are surrounded by so many that are very worried about what others may think about them, but the reality is people are too busy worrying about themselves to worry about you too. Do you and be you and applaud others for doing the same.

The greatest failures have led to the greatest successes. In the past two weeks I have interviewed two people on The Jason and Pili Project podcast who combined have lost over $100 Million Dollars. If they spent all their time worrying about what other people thought of them, they would never have come back to make multiples of that and help thousands along the way.

#3) Not knowing why I really want what I want...

I hear this constantly – random statements about wishes and wants. What's missing is an actual reason you want it. Our minds are wired to find the easiest route. The road to a better life has speed bumps and if we aren't painfully specific about why we want what we want, our mind will always lead us back to the safest route that will leave us where we are.

#4) Negative talk track from those close to you ...

Here's the hard truth. Your wants may be different from your loved ones…. That doesn't mean they don't love you or you have to cut them out of your life.

The reality is that if you are a person who wants big, gigantic, unrelenting greatness in your life, you stand alone in a field where the rest of the world hasn't found that need and doesn't understand that want.

If you want it, go get it. Your loved ones don't shut you down to hurt you; they just can't grasp the magnitude of what you are doing and say what they say because they think they are protecting you.

When you get what you want in life, I guarantee their words will change and they will miraculously find support in what you do.

Action Step:

Identify what's stopping you and give it a name like Bob or Betty. Now every time you get in a position where you might talk or think yourself out of doing what needs to be done, say "Not today Betty! Today is for doing and I am getting it done."

DAY 9:
BUILD YOUR FOUNDATION

"A house must be built on solid foundations if it is to last. The same principle applies to man, otherwise he too will sink back into the soft ground and become swallowed up by the world of illusion." - Sai Baba

On Day 5 we identified where we are and what brings us joy in each space. Now is time to build the path to what each space with represent next.

Here are the five best ways to start charting your new course:

1. Jot down all the main buckets in your life. This may include family, relationships, work, fitness, hobbies or a number of different items.
2. Set the major focuses for each bucket. For family, it may be spending quality time together, or for fitness, it may be doing four thirty-minute workouts a week.
3. Label what your current life looks like and how you are attending to each of the buckets.
4. Identify what right now an ideal setting for each of those buckets would be.
5. Set a priority and hierarchy for each of the buckets. This may be allocated to certain seasons or certain times of years.

6. Implement the plan. Now that the plan is defined, use it as your foundation for all your decision making. Not only will this allow clarity for your future, but also it will define your next steps forward.

Remember, creating a life plan is like setting a road map for where you want to go. Sometimes there is a detour but you have the destination set. Identifying a new work experience or new employment opportunity may be a priority. A road map isn't just about your current or past employment history, or your work experience, or your salary – it's what your future looks like and who you want to be.

If you feel like you've done everything right up to this point, write down a plan for what's next. Here's a list of major areas of your life you might want to focus on: career, health, finances, relationship, and happiness. Identify yourself as the person you want to be, and make a list of things you can do to make that a reality. Make this plan solid and sticky and make it part of who you are.

Don't know where to start? That's ok. Anything right now is better than nothing. I start with the first thing that comes to mind.

If you want to be a dentist, what would that do for your time, finances, family and health? If you want to lose 20 pounds, what would that do for your energy, time, relationships and outlook on life? There's no wrong starting place. The only wrong move is to do nothing at all.

Know your goals, get them nailed down, and set structure around where you want to be. Make it clear to everyone around you that you have plans for the future, and they'll be more likely to follow along the journey with you.

Now that you're on a path to take, it's time to act on it.

Work on the fundamentals, because they are the foundation for everything else. This includes prioritizing your time, finding and keeping your focus, and finding strong connections that help you make even more connections that propel you forward in your progress.

A Few Areas of Focus:

Exercise - Strength, flexibility and health is key to a sustained life.

Meditate - This really makes you more peaceful and happier, and helps you clearly think about the challenges and worries you have, as well as how you can handle them.

Eat a healthy diet – This helps keep you feeling energized and focused, helps you maintain your sanity and focus, and helps you to be healthy and happy.

Volunteer – These volunteer things may seem a little trivial, but they can add up to a big difference in your life, and can do wonders for your ability to focus and stay on task.

If there are any areas that you struggle with, then I would encourage you to just focus on those things and use them to get better.

So, next time you struggle with anything in life, you can take a step back and look at how you can manage your thoughts and focus in a better way. You may just find yourself getting a lot more done in your life, and improving all the time.

Do you struggle with any problems related to your thoughts? Have you ever tried any of these methods?

There may be detours and flat tires along the way, but having a map to the destination will always allow you to find your way back to the path.

ACTION STEP:

For the next five days do: 5 minutes of any exercise, 5 minutes of meditation, make a 5-minute call to your doctor or nutritionist or a mentor or educator and donate 5 dollars to a charity or give 5 minutes of time to help someone in need 'without' asking if they need help. Did you know you can start a donation thread on Facebook and let your friends donate as well?! Then

DAY 10:
SURROUND YOURSELF WITH POSITIVITY

Positivity starts with you! Surround yourself within! Do not let others or your environment dictate your mindset. YOU CHOOSE.

I (Pili) didn't always have this way of being. I let myself be dictated to. Here is a conversation I had with the old me...

I look fairly healthy. I have always been skinny and fit. I write a health and wellness blog. What could possibly be wrong?

But eight Summers ago, I was anorexic.

Let Me introduce you to Me.

Here's a conversation between my old me (PN) and the new me (PY)...

Pili Nathaniel (8 years ago): (PN) "I was anorexic."

Pili Yarusi (PY): "WAIT FOR ME TO ASK THE QUESTION!!! First, how would you describe yourself for the folks?"

PN: "Now? I am a healthy and happy thirty-two-year-old Hawaiian-ish woman, and my many ethnicities would fill this page. I am a woman currently living with my parents in Mililani, Hawaii. That sounds depressing but it is what I needed. Their love guided me through some pretty tough times."

PY: "How did you find out that you had an eating disorder?"

PN: "Once I got back to my parents' house, I finally went to a doctor. She did a complete checkup and blood work. She knew I was underweight by just looking at me. At that moment I was 112 lbs. I am 5'8". According to the Center of Disease and Control, anywhere between 122-164 lbs. would be considered healthy. I then explained my difficulties prior how I was trying to overcome them."

PY: "You said, 'At that MOMENT...' How much did you weigh before?"

PN: "I started losing weight at a very rapid rate from about May into September (2012). I had nothing really to lose in the first place. I lost about twenty pounds. The lowest that I checked was 105 lbs."

PY: "Shit."

PN: "Yeah. I used to weigh myself ALL THE TIME. I got kinda obsessed about it. I knew something was wrong, but I didn't know what and I was too scared to see a doctor. I'm pretty sure that's the lowest."

PY: "Didn't anyone say anything?"

PN: "Yeah. All the time. One of my friends mothers even asked me point blank, "Pili, are you anorexic? You don't look healthy. I know you have always been skinny... but right now, you look sick."

That's pretty close to her exact words. I told her that I was fine and that I was eating. She didn't say anything more. My good friends behind the bar would ask me if I was okay and I'd basically just brush them off. They kept me functioning, though. I'd find snickers bars and snacks at my register. My manager even started to order my food for me... or at least he'd make sure I wasn't just eating a salad. So yeah... people said things. I just chose not to hear."

PY: "Your coworkers sound awesome... (that coworker was Jason btw!) ... Why do you think you got this way?"

PN: "My doctor said the anorexia was brought on by depression."

PY: "Depression? You want to elaborate?"

PN: "No."

PY: "Hmm...ok. Have you seen a therapist or any specialists?"

PN: "No. I probably should. But by my next appointment with her two weeks later, I'd been in LA and SF for about a week, I had gained five pounds and was at 121 lbs. and holding. She saw that I was already taking care of myself and on the road to recovery. She told me then that she thought I'd been anorexic due to the depression. She also said that she had not seen such amazing charts in a long time. She said everything was clean and healthy except for the extreme weight loss and that I was hypoglycemic. It was probably triggered by anorexia, she said."

PY: "Please explain..."

PN: "It basically means I have a tendency towards having low blood sugar. Normal blood sugar is anywhere between 70 – 100. I was at 40. She said that she would normally refer me to specialists and a therapist but that she thought MY FAMILY and SUPPORTIVE FRIENDS were doing the job."

PY: "How did you begin to CHANGE YOUR LIFE and EAT HEALTHY again?"

PN: "That is exactly what I did. I chose to be HAPPY. I moved back in with my family. I began EATING again... and eating as MUCH as I wanted. My doctor friend in New York told me that my calorie intake, just to keep my body functioning at 5'8", 105 lbs., was 1,300 calories. He said that I was probably only taking in on average 1,000 calories. I put myself on an app called Calorie Counter and made sure my intake was at least 1,800-2,000 a day. Calorie Counter is still trying to get me to be 144 lbs., but I don't think that's going to happen. I stepped up my exercise routine. I worked with a personal trainer for about two weeks. Instead of just yoga, I added cardio and strength training."

PY: "How much do you weigh?"

PN: "This morning I weighed 126 lbs. I could stand to gain a few more but this is my NORMAL HEALTHY weight."

...

OKAAAY... enough of that. I gotta stop talking to myself. You might start thinking I'm crazy or something. However, in all seriousness, if you think that you or someone you know may have an eating disorder, talk to them. Show your support and love for them. Urge them to SEE A DOCTOR. Get a physical. Get a checkup. Even if they do not have an eating disorder there may be something else wrong.

For continued reading here's some information on Eating Disorders:

Anorexia (Mayo Clinic Staff): "Anorexia nervosa is an eating disorder that causes people to obsess about their weight and the food they eat. People with anorexia nervosa attempt to maintain a weight that's far below normal for their age and height. To prevent weight gain or to continue losing weight, people with anorexia nervosa may starve themselves or exercise excessively.

Anorexia (an-oh-REK-see-uh) nervosa isn't really about food. It's an unhealthy way to try to cope with emotional problems. When you have anorexia nervosa, you often equate thinness with self-worth.

Anorexia nervosa can be difficult to overcome. But with treatment, you can gain a better sense of who you are, return to healthier eating habits and reverse some of anorexia's serious complications."

The first step in promoting a healthy and positive life for yourself is to first MAKE THE DECISION. It is your choice to CHOOSE HAPPINESS and POSITIVITY. Pain happens and we all deal with it differently. But suffering is OPTIONAL.

You need to decide to stand up for yourself and to fill your life with positive influences. That's what I did. You can too.

Here are some small steps:

This can be much harder to manage. Please remember these two things:

Make it a point to reach out to others every day. Talk to those you love and who love you for YOU – EVERY FREAKING DAY! Connect with at least one person daily – an old friend, a business acquaintance or a family member. We need to put forth the effort in order to see real change and love in a person. Do not wait for those you love to extend their hand. They might be needing you to extend yours.

And...

Just because someone is family or has been in your life for a time DOESN'T mean they get to be toxic. You can give them grace but there will come a time that you will bend so much that you will break. That is not fair to you or the loved ones that do care about you and your wellbeing.

Social Media: "I saw something that I didn't agree with online. I kept scrolling through instead of engaging and wasn't bothered." There are many ways to stop negativity from entering your mind from the internet.

Limit yourself. We strive to disconnect during family times and evenings. Set these "No Social Media" times in your calendar and stick to them.

Stop Scrolling. Pili only checks notifications and groups we love and manage. Scrolling becomes a mindless adventure in time-suckery.

Use the Block and Mute features of social media. Many apps have ways you can block or mute people in your "social media circle." Filter out those who are negative. You don't need that in your life.

Surround yourself with positivity! Follow those who have a mindset and attitude you want to emulate. "Success leaves clues!" The more you surround yourself with the type of success you want, the more likely you will receive it!

HOW TO MASTER A FIT RICH LIFE IN 15 DAYS! | 61

Action Step:

Take 10 minutes to review one of your Social Media hangouts. Does your feed exude the confidence and strength you are looking to achieve? Is it filled with success and extraordinary people? Is it filled with the light and happiness that you crave? You choose what you see... Fix your social media accordingly. This will take a few days or months to correct. You do not need other people's BS filtering into your mind!

DAY 11:
GO BEYOND YOUR BOUNDARIES

Find accountability whether through others or within yourself.

Hey – Jason here again. I always tried to do it myself. I always thought, why would I need anyone else's help? I was too proud and honestly too weak to open up about the actual help I needed. The real truth is all of my major growth has happened once I learned to open myself up to others. It made me accountable and although I was uncomfortable, it allowed me to peel back another layer and get real with what it is that I actually needed.

This can be hard but doing hard things is what morphs us into the person we are meant to become.

A simple way to begin to overcome excuses is taking very small action steps. Say "Yes" the very next time your immediate reaction is to say "No." The next time you feel the urge to say "I CAN'T," adjust your wording to, "I WILL!" While these may seem like small adjustments, the massive positive byproducts of these changes will have a colossal impact on your outlook on life.

Once you have mastered this, and you *can* and *will* master this, start changing little things in your day to just prove to yourself you are tougher than you think. This will also push you to realize how great you have it.

Skip breakfast for three straight days. Take a cold shower for 5 consecutive nights or sleep on the floor for a week straight. Wake up at 3 am for 5 straight days. Why do this? Because you can. Do this to prove to yourself how tough you can be when you choose to and after that 3rd day sleeping on the wooden floor, you will truly appreciate and cherish that fourth day back in your comfy bed, being able to sleep till 6:30 am or taking a warm shower. These moments will start your journey and propel you to say "Yes" to what terrified you before.

I wake up at 4:32AM. That's a memorable time, right? When asked, "What time do you wake up?", I tell them that I live by the 4-3-2-1 Principle. I wake up at 4:32AM and I beat the sun out of bed each day, so that makes me number 1, and it's my first win of the day. What can you create that's memorable in your daily habits?

When I first decided to run The New York City Marathon, I couldn't even run a mile. I hadn't ever run for distance and the thought of running 26.2 miles was not one I could mentally grasp. After months of training and commitment, I completed the race in 3 hours and 50 minutes. I enjoyed the race that day which taught me a valuable lesson.

First, I could have pushed harder – I had played it safe. I had set my goals too low and had not given myself enough expectations. I think a lot of us do this. We assume we can't, so we set the bar low to not be disappointed.

Second, the mental barrier leading up to the race far exceeded the physical exertion. This served to be a tremendous lesson some 9 years later when I ran my first 100-mile race. A few months prior to the 100-mile race was the first time I had heard about ultra-running. Instead of doing what I had done prior for marathons and doing a running program, I chose to focus solely on willing my mind to know I can run 100 miles. I had never run even close to that in a single day. I knew the real challenge would be to not let my mind take over and distort my outcome by convincing my body that what I was doing could not be done. They say when our mind tries to give up, our body is only at 40% and sometimes we just have to remind ourselves of that.

I ran daily between 5-7 miles and did a few 15 and 20 mile runs and the day of the race I told myself that it was already done before I started and told my mind I was just here to get to the end and pick up my belt buckle (the award for finishing the race in 24 hours or less – I did it in 21 hours). That talk track served me well that day and I continue to use the narrative today. Know your limits fall on you and only you can stop yourself.

(Pili here now...)

I entered a race called TOUGH MUDDER. I had All the Excuses NOT to do this one...

It. Was. Crazy.

So crazy that I think my brain went numb in the Mason Container ice-bath and I just couldn't write about it. I couldn't think about it. Even now I tremble with delighted FEAR at the prospect of ever doing it again.

So that brain-numbing sphincter-clenching TOUGH MUDDER was so... Well... Let me take you through some of my favorite parts of the course. Let's go with:

PILI'S TOP TEN TOUGH MUDDER HIGHLIGHTS

or better known as…

HOW PILI GOT HER ASS KICKED!

10. *The Running*. I am going to admit it here. I was the last one on my team to EVERY obstacle. Between my timidness, my lack of stamina, and my need to conserve energy I just SUCKED when it came to pumping myself up to run. Even though my teammates kept up a good pace, I could not stay in time with them. I don't like admitting this. I trained for three months to get myself into running shape.

9. *The Cold*. I hate being cold. I knew this was coming. I thought I could handle it. By the end of the race I could barely hold my beer because I was shaking so hard.

8. *The Shower*. Almost the hardest part of the whole thing. ARE YOU KIDDING ME?!!! After three HARD hours in crazy obstacle-course land I had to wash off in an ICY shower.

7. *Fatigue*. I not only trained to run; I also trained my body to take the hardships that were dealt in the TOUGH MUDDER… at least that is what I thought. I really felt like the weak link. I did not have the massive strength needed to really be a key player.

6. *Funky Monkey*. Yeah… This obstacle is basically a set of Monkey Bars on ACID. I made it to the first bar

and slipped off. Regular monkey bars are hard enough as it is… Add wet mud. Hard!

5. *Arctic Enema.* Imagine jumping into a pool filled with ice cubes and muddy water. Imagine swimming though this pool and then dunking your head under the ice-cube-water for three seconds – and then swimming for another ten. That wasn't the hard part. The hard part was trying to climb out when your entire body is screaming because your muscles were locking up...

4. *All those Walls.* The short ones. The tall ones. Ranging from 5ft to 30ft (It looked like 30ft to me!). Wow. It looked like there was just no way.

3. *Electroshock Therapy.* Nothing more needs to be said.

2. Mud Mile. This is toward the end of the course. It includes HILLS OF MUD, WALLS OF MUD, DEEP POOLS OF COLD MUDDY WATER and MORE MUD.

1. I know I mentioned this before – the RUNNING KILLED ME.

BUT…

I would do it all again.

Why?

Because I FINISHED. I COMPLETED ALL THE OBSTACLES. I did not "opt out." I did not freeze and cry at the top of the 30ft tower. (It was probably closer to 15ft) I JUMPED OFF!!! It was exhilarating! It felt good to overcome my fears. It felt amazing to feel PAIN. To feel like I could fall on my face at any moment. To feel angry at myself for not pushing harder.

How did I do this?

Teammates.

Their names were Jason, Christina, Ben, Adam and the countless people I ran with who helped push me along by running alongside me, helping me up, showing me where to go and allowing me to help them as well.

I know in the beginning I said I was the weak link... I was. BUT I STILL SUPPORTED MY TEAM and in TURN THEY SUPPORTED ME. I am very thankful to all of them for showing me that I can do these crazy things. They gave me a shoulder to lean on... or climb on... in this case!

Here's to HEALTH and MUD!

ACTION STEPS:

Strive to be uncomfortable and say yes to what you have been saying no to.

Want to be a writer and don't know where to start? Just start writing the first ten words that you can think of right now.

Want to start a business? Write in a Facebook forum or Reddit group, where no one you know will be, and speak about the viability of your business.

Want to make a new product? Write 8 words that will describe how you as the customer will feel using this product.

Want to buy real estate? Write 5 words for what buying real estate means to you.

Want to run in a Tough Mudder or a Marathon – go sign up for the next one!

Make your choice and do this right now....

I'm waiting for you to get it done!

The longer you wait to do these tasks, no matter how small, the more likely it won't get done. And are these tasks really small? If you haven't taken action in five years, then the truth is these tasks are massive!

This can be the pinnacle moment driving you forward. You are here to find fulfillment. If none of the above resonates with you, then write 6 things that interest you or 5 things you like to eat or 7 types of workouts you like or even write 5 things we could have done better in this book. Trust us when we say this – we seek daily to be uncomfortable and soliciting feedback is one of the best ways for us to learn and move forward. If you choose the latter, text us your feedback to +1 (908) 224-6876. You will not hurt our feelings! The goal here is to step outside your comfort zone today. Not tomorrow.

DAY 12:
MAKE EXCUSES PAY

"The way to get started is to quit talking and begin doing."
– Walt Disney

When you come up with an excuse, notice it, accept and label it, and tell it that it isn't welcome any longer. Look for EXCUSE PATTERNS and repeat to yourself, *"It's time to be a difference maker."*

We all have our comfort zone and the area where we feel safe. However, times have softened our safety zone. Centuries ago decisions were made daily in the context of will this help me "eat, sleep and survive". The basic human instincts created the sense of stress we still feel today. Now times are a different version of tough. We don't have those saber-toothed tigers chasing us, but we still get that distressed feeling as the fight or flight nature is still inbred into our DNA.

So how do we change this narrative?

First, identify the excuse. What is it that you say or do when something happens that will potentially push you outside of your comfort zone? Do you manifest a heightened sense of urgency in times where there is no great risk to your wellbeing?

Is there a saber-toothed tiger chasing you?

It's time to excuse yourself from your excuses and let them know you aren't coming back. Tell them that you're breaking up with them and their ways no longer fits your life and mindset. They no longer fit who you are, who you want to be and who you are becoming.

Repeat this *"I am a difference maker.* When tough times come, I look for the solution. I look at a problem as a task to conquer, not as an issue. Today I no longer have an excuse; I have a way forward."

Excuses don't fit in your life. Do you want to be known as the person who always says "...but?" Well here's your chance to go "Men In Black" on your excuses and permanently erase them from your memory, your self-talk and your life.

Make the decision right now that today, you no longer make excuses. You find solutions. If you have an excuse in front of you for something you want to accomplish, you need to ask yourself, "Is this something I want in my life or is it something that just sounds good to me and I don't need it?" If it's the latter, erase it from your memory as it's something you don't need to be doing.

Warren Buffet has a 5/25 rule. He writes down 25 things he wants to accomplish in the foreseeable future and then ranks them in order of importance and circles the top 5 on the list. He then avoids all twenty that he didn't circle until he's conquered the top 5. Buffet says, "No matter what, these things get no attention from you until you've succeeded with your top 5."

It's time to get working and excuses that aren't needed are no longer welcome here. Telling your excuses "you're not welcome here" helps – telling them "get out of my head!"

helps more. And making a stand that "I no longer negotiate with myself, under any circumstances" is the true, final statement. The stand starts now. It's time to take on the excuses you make and get things done. So let's get to work.

I (Jason) used to be the king of excuses. I remember one day in high school where I had walked into English class late for over the tenth time in a month and handed the teacher a note with the reason _other_ on it. The teacher finally noticed and then he asked, "What are all these 'others' for being late?" The truth was, there was no good truth besides I was being lazy and not taking responsibility for being on time and I was a wizard at crafting tales to circumvent this.

It wasn't until years later that I realized that skirting the truth once is the same as doing it a dozen times. How you do anything will be how you do everything. If you want greatness, then you have to show up and be responsible – not just today, but every day. I stopped being late by making "being on time" a priority. I get what's needed to be done, even if it means waking up two hours early or staying up three hours late. I eat clean and have cleaned up my drinking, even if it makes me miss parties where my interests no longer align or not celebrate in the same fashion as everyone else. And while this may have raised eyebrows, this is what I had to do for myself. I had to show up as my authentic self no matter where I was, and no matter what I was doing.

ACTION STEPS:

Today, when an excuse comes up, find the positive rebuttal to it. This should be the furthest thing or exact opposite from what that excuse is telling you. This way, "I don't have time" becomes "I have all the time in the world." "I can't make it to my daughter's recital" becomes "I can't wait to attend more." "I keep making bad business decisions" becomes "I am learning so much about what it takes to become successful." Or, "My wife and I keep disagreeing" becomes "I'm ready to find more ways to agree."

Next, find the bridge. Don't have time? Well, make the event you don't have time for the pinnacle moment of your day. Force yourself to find the time to get all the things you told yourself you needed to do done. If they are that important, you will accomplish them.

DAY 13:
BE OBSESSED WITH GREATNESS

*"People Who Are Crazy Enough To Think They Can
Change The World, Are The Ones Who Do."*
– Rob Siltanen

You deserve your best self, your best life and your best future.

We all have greatness in us – we just need to stop telling ourselves we don't.

Where do you get off not being great? You're reading this book so you want it, but, the actual truth is you already have it. Just let your mind get out of the way. Our minds have habits of tricking us into averages and poor routines. It's easier for the mind. Easier for you too. But the easy thing to do is be average. So, take yourself out of your comfort zone. Do things that test you.

At first, going towards excellence may be difficult, but why not try it? Can't figure it out? Then go pick up the phone and call the most successful person you can think of and ask "how do you do it?" Or, go on Instagram and DM ten highly successful people and ask them "what has been the key to your greatness?" We're waiting!

Remember, a great life is a fulfilled life. When we use the term greatness, that doesn't just mean the richest person you know. We know plenty of people who have a ton of money and are miserable and we know a ton of people who don't and never stop smiling. Find what greatness means to you. To me (Jason), greatness is showing up as a great father, husband and business partner and doing the little things that I know makes a difference when no one's looking, like, putting the grocery cart back at the supermarket. Trust me, expect greatness from yourself and don't settle for less. Show up like a champion and create your greatness simply by letting it finally shine through.

Here are reasons why you may not be able to let greatness in:

1. You keep comparing yourself to others, without knowing their full story.
2. You attribute too much of your journey to the opinions of others.
3. You will not start until you are perfectly ready.
4. You focus on the word "Greatness" without actually identifying what that means to you.
5. You determine your goal and go for it without making a plan for the first actionable step and then quit when the first hurdle comes up.
6. You assume it's going to be tough, so you tell yourself you'll start tomorrow, then next week, then the week after and then never start.
7. You think greatness is the final achievement and the rest of your days will be set when it's just the first step in the journey.

It is your responsibility to CHOOSE GREATNESS! How many times do you find yourself reliving horrible moments in your life? How many times in the day do you automatically think negatively? Do you play the blame game? Do you BLAME others for events in your life, good and bad? SURE. We ALL do. But we can stop the circle of negative thought – negative thoughts that inhibit our growth potential. We can stop by allowing ourselves FIVE MINUTES to be ANGRY, NEGATIVE, SPITEFUL, DOWN, DEPRESSED, SHIT ON, AMBIVALENT, SAD... and my favorite, CRABBY. You have five minutes.

Think about something negative. Start small. Do you have your something? Good. Now for five minutes, let yourself feel what you need to feel. Blame your husband, mom, dad, roommate... Blame the world for your misfortune. Be in that moment. You have FIVE MINUTES.

Now stop. Now it is UP TO YOU to take RESPONSIBILITY for that event. No matter what happened, it is up to YOU to take responsibility for YOUR REACTION. You can either let it inhibit your growth, or you can grow past it. IT HAPPENED... THERE IS NOTHING YOU CAN DO ABOUT IT NOW. Take responsibility and MOVE FORWARD! Whether forward means correcting a situation, moving on, letting go or whatever... Do what you need to do to live a HAPPY LIFE... a life of fulfillment... a life worth living.

ACTION STEPS:

Go the extra step the next time you can. Be Great in small ways.

Examples:

- Send a thank you note in the mail.

- Pick Up Trash when out and about, even if it's not your mess.

- Go out of your way to thank someone.

DAY 14:
YOU ARE ENOUGH!

No matter where you start or where you get to, it will always be enough. Knowing your true self is truly the fulfilling prophecy.

A few months ago I (Jason) did a running challenge called the Calendar Club. You run the mile of each day of the month. Day 1 you run 1 mile, day 15 you run 15 miles and day 30 you run 30 miles. It was a total of 465 miles in a 30 day month.

It wasn't easy but honestly would it have been worth it if it was?

It was physical, but even more mental.

Here's the parallel to our life.

How many times have we talked ourselves out of doing something even when we knew it was good for us? I should eat better, workout more, call my mother, learn this skill that could help me get a job I actually love or I should meet new friends. But somehow our mind tricks us into not doing these things out of fear of the unknown and back to "stuck in the same place" we go.

How many times have you thought about doing something, but paralyzed yourself by thinking of all the negative possibilities that could happen? When you think of possibilities for an outcome, how many are bad and how many are good? I would bet that most are potentially horrible results. The truth is in almost every scenario if you do venture out and try, it may not go as planned, but the worst-case scenario rarely happens.

So why do we think this way? Well it's easier. That's it.

We are prone to think of every hole in the story. Try telling someone around you about your dreams and aspirations and they will pick them apart trying to give you every counter and caveat. Rarely will you hear "give it a go." Well, you will now, because in the chapter for day 10, you chose to surround yourself with positivity and people looking for the solutions. This is why iron-cladding your mind and surrounding yourself with positivity is fundamental in your journey. It's great to have close ones and loved ones, but sometimes you need to keep them in your life and find another outlet to find your positivity.

Your close ones may not be prepared, yet, for your journey. And one thing we do know is that we cannot change others until they are ready, open and willing for change. Change starts with them – the same as positive change made now by you.

So, how do we get past this hurdle – past this constant reminder of how "easier would be better" and where "safer" is better just because it seems more comfortable?

It starts again with words "I Will", "I am", and "I Can."

Sounds simple right? But what if we changed our wording to meet what our actions will be? No longer shall we allow ourselves to use "I Should" or "Maybe I can," because you are no longer going to be yesterday's version of you.

Doing this may sound minimal. But small constant steps go a long way. So, today is the time to course correct – to set you on a course not only to achieve what you were set here to do, but also to give you a base to fall back on when your mind tells you, "It's OK to eat that Twinkie."

Remember, nothing worth having comes easy. The more you align and train your mind to know this is "Who You Are Now", the easier it will be when doubt and fear come into play.

Don't worry about being scared. Fear shows that you care and that what you are doing has meaning.

Meryl Streep still gets stage fright. She is known as one of the greatest actresses ever, but her mind tries to limit her from being great... "Just come back to average," her mind tries to implore. The difference is making the decision to push through because "I Will," "I Am," and "I Can."

It's not always your mind that will try to limit you. It may be your tribe or your surroundings or even your shoes. As I (Jason) started the 22nd day of running, where I had to run 22 miles, my shoes decided that it was no longer something they wanted to be a part of and so my toes broke completely through the right shoe.

Back on day 16, I had one hole in the shoe and on day 20 a second hole formed. These are shoes that had trekked some 1,000 plus miles. But "I can and will" was in my head and there was no excuse that was going to stop me. My shoes had no choice but to suck it up and accompany me to the end of my journey!

Action Steps:

Today continues to bring new challenges and tomorrow will too. Just keep "will"ing and "can"ing. No more average. No more complacency. Just action.

Today, right now, text us at **+1 (908) 224-6876** and let us know a goal that you accomplished that no one thought you could attain. We will celebrate your win with you.

Know you are, were and continue to be enough.

Let's do this!

DAY 15:
CONGRATULATING YOUR
FUTURE SELF

See yourself today as the person you truly want to be. Find what it is that defines your win. Dance crazy. Shake your toosh! Pound your chest. Roar loud…

Find meaning in understanding, WHAT YOUR FUTURE SELF WILL NO LONGER TOLERATE…

If you are like me (Pili), you have a hard time taking a moment to look at where you were and where you are today. There is nothing more important than taking a moment for you and your success. Now, this isn't a go out and get stupid kind of moment, but this is a moment to take the space to observe yourself. Who you are and what you are doing now is massively important. This needs to be passed on not only for you, but to your partner, your children, your associates or your teammates.

What you have to offer is invaluable and irreplaceable. Reflect and give your mind the space to prepare for what's ahead. I like to do this each morning, as we spoke about in earlier chapters. I find if I can take the time for me first, it allows me to start the day with clarity and with a clean perspective. For the days that I don't get this time, it's like trying to jump on a moving freight train.

ACTION STEPS:

Success Comes In All Shapes, Colors and Sizes and at Any Age...

<u>Over the next 15 days:</u> Note your daily successes. For Day 15, write what your full list of successes will be as if you are looking back and have already accomplished them.

Now, do this for your larger goals as if it was 5 years from now by doing the following:

Get some paper and a pen.

1. Add five years to today's date. Write that date at the top of the paper.

2. In very specific detail, write down every part of that day – the smells and the weather – where you are and what you are doing. What time did you wake up? Who are you with? Write down the feelings and emotions that you have...

3. It is important to understand that the work you put in TODAY will allow you to have what you want in the future. Make every part of this future date as detailed as possible. The power is in the detail.

4. And finally, please share with us at +1 (908) 224-6876!

You now have the key to building accomplishment into your day and learning winning habits. Most of us have let ourselves off the hook for years. But now, instead, determine in your mind RIGHT NOW is the time.

Make your bed as soon as you get up in the morning. Cook all your meals on Sunday night so you are prepped for the whole week. Open doors for others. Say "Thank You." Pick up after yourself. Pick up after others. Make the call that needs to be made, and always tell the truth.

Any of these actions will continue training your mind that you are back and this time you are here to win. Make your day a series of wins so when the next big test comes, you only know how to win.

Be specific with who you are and who you will be. This isn't the time to sugarcoat it with yourself. That didn't work and won't work. It's just one more step to getting to the "you" that looks at tests as learning experiences and not let downs. The difference between winning and losing is the winners will risk losing more than the losers will ever try.

Winners win the moment and build momentum to get to the big goal in front of them. They stop the ball at the top of the hill, position it correctly and then push it down the road and let the buildup of energy carry them forward…

CONCLUSION

This is your life. You get to choose to create whatever kind of life that you really, truly want. The question then is, what do you really want and what is the best way to get there?

It is our belief that these 15 steps or days of action towards your goals are what is going to make all the difference in the world for you. It did for us! And it will for you too...

Here is a road map laid out for you but you need to step out on the road to start the journey. No one big step will do it but small, every day, gradual, progressive steps will build the life you desire. Not every day will be perfect but why would you want it that way anyway? This way, when those perfect days show up more and more, you will truly appreciate them to their fullest.

Thank you so much for taking the time to read our book! It was a lot of fun for us to create this and share it with you. We sincerely hope that you take us up on our offer to text us what transformations you have made since the start of this book at +1 (908) 224-6876.

From both of our hearts, Jason and Pili,

Aloha!

Now, Let's Do This!